My Healthy Lean and Green Cookbook for Meat and Fish dishes

50 affordable and super easy meat and fish recipes for your lean and green diet to stay healthy and boost energy

Josephine Reed

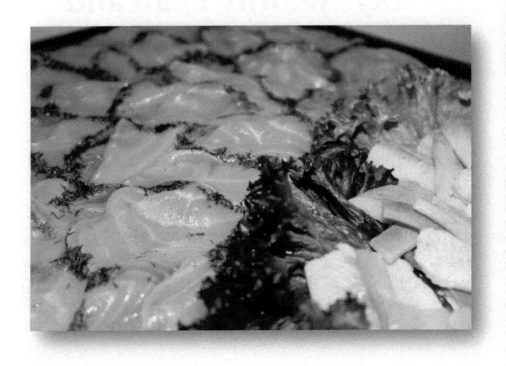

Table of contents

Garlic Crusted Flank Steak with Roasted Tomato Relish 8

Seafood & Scallions Creole 11

Sweet & Smoky Pulled Chicken 13

Garlic Crusted BBQ Baby Back Ribs.. 15

Juicy Rosemary Pulled Pork... 17

Slow-Cooked Chicken with Fire Roasted Tomatoes 19

Finger Licking BBQ Crock Pot Chicken................................... 21

Big Mac in a Bowl.. 23

Coconut Flour Chicken Nuggets 25

Skinny Chicken Salad 27

Chicken Marsala... 29

Turkey Meatloaf... 32

Chicken Piccata 35

Chicken, Bell Pepper & Carrot Curry....................................... 37

Chicken Chili 39

Beef and Kale Casserole... 41

Beef and Mushroom Soup 43

Salmon with cucumbers, tomatoes, and dill salad.................... 45

Salmon burgers with cucumber salad 47

Roasted red pepper sauce scallops and zucchini noodles......... 49

Stir-fried winter melon with shrimp 51

Roasted lemon pepper salmon and garlic Parmesan asparagus 53

Avocado lime shrimp salad... 55

Steamed Seafood Pot...56

Avocado lime tuna salad...58

Low-carb lobster roll 59

Noodle soup...61

Steamed white fish street tacos 64

Stir-fry shrimps with champignon mushroom and broccoli.....66

Steamed stuffed mushrooms (with pork) 68

Sheet pan shrimp scampi 70

Sambal Kang Kong with bay scallops.........................72

Crab and asparagus frittata..75

Shrimp and cauliflower grits......................................77

Zucchini sheet with shrimp and scampi 79

Crab zucchini sushi rolls 81

Oyster omelet..83

Spicy crab stuffed avocado 85

Blackened shrimp lettuce wraps 87

Beef & Veggies Stew..89

Beef & Carrot Chili..92

Beef & Carrot Curry 94

Pork Lettuce Wraps 96

Chicken Alfredo Pesto Pasta 98

Chicken Pesto Paninis 100

Chicken With Ginger Pesto 101

Creamy Pesto Chicken...103

Keto Lobster Roll But With Crab 105

Salmon with Veggies 107

Baked cod with tomatoes and feta..109

Garlic Crusted Flank Steak with Roasted Tomato Relish

Prep Time: 5 mi and 1 h refrigerate

Cook Time: 25 min

Serve: 6

Ingredients:

- Steak
- 2 tablespoons chopped fresh thyme
- 2 normal spoons chopped fresh rosemary 1 tablespoon chopped fresh tarragon
- 2 garlic cloves, minced 2 teaspoons salt.
- 1 ½ little spoons ground black-pepper 2 1 ½ pound flank steaks
- 1 tablespoon olive oil Tomatoes
- 2 cups halved cherry tomatoes
- 1 cup chopped fresh Italian parsley
- 1/4 cup of Kalamata pitted olives coarsely chopped or other black olives brine-cured
- ¼ cup coarsely-chopped pitted green olives with brine-cured
- 1/4 cup chopped new basil

8

- 1/4 cup of extra virgin olive oil
- 2 tablespoons Sherry wine vinegar

Instructions:

1.Preheat oven to 375 degrees F.

2. Process the tomatoes in a food processor until smooth. Pulse the beef herbs into the sprigs, along with the garlic, salt, and pepper, until the mixture is finely chopped and the herbs are gone. Drizzle in the olive oil with the engine running. The relish can be made, covered, and refrigerated a day in advance.

3.On a work surface, lay the steaks out side by side. Spoon a third of the relish over the steaks, spread it over the meat with a spatula, and be careful not to tear it. Sprinkle with the herb-garlic mixture and roll up the steaks lengthwise. Place them and drizzle them with olive oil in a baking dish. Let stand at room temperature for 30 minutes.

4.Roast the steaks for 10 minutes. Turn them and continue roasting until medium-rare (135 degrees F) or medium (140 degrees F), about 10 minutes more. The steaks can rest up to 10 minutes before slicing.

5.In a bowl, to make the tomatoes, toss together the tomatoes, herbs, olives, and basil with the vinegar and oil; season to taste with salt and pepper.

6.Cut the steak rolls crosswise on the diagonal into 1 1/2-inch-thick slice. Serve the steak between the tomato slices.

Nutrition: Energy (calories): 2236 kcal Protein: 334.68 g Fat: 84.92 g Carbohydrates: 10.36 g Calcium, Ca372 mg Magnesium, Mg359 mg Phosphorus, P3165 mg

Seafood & Scallions Creole

Prep Time: 10 minutes

Cook Time: 30 minutes

Serve: 5

Ingredients:

- 4 regular butter spoons 1 big onion, diced 1 celery rib, diced
- 1 green bell pepper, 2 cloves of garlic, 1/2 teaspoon of thyme salt, 1/2 teaspoon of thyme salt
- One-half teaspoon black pepper
- ½ teaspoon cayenne pepper 1 Tablespoon flour
- 1/3 cup dry white wine (optional)
- 1 15 oz of tomatoes or around 1 1/4 cups of fresh tomatoes peeled and diced
- 1 cup stock of chicken, 2 bay leaves
- 2 lb of spicy pepper sauce, such as Tabasco, to taste. Oh, huge uncooked shrimp (about 32)
- For serving, 6-8 cups of hot cooked rice
- 2 green onions for garnish, sliced,

Instructions:

1.In a big saucepan or Dutch oven, heat 2 tablespoons of the butter over medium-high. Add the onion, celery, bell pepper, and garlic and cook stirring, until softened, about 3 minutes.

2.Ad the shrimp and cook, stirring, until they just turn pink, about 2 minutes. Stir in the salt, thyme, black pepper, and cayenne.

3.Stir in the remaining 2 normal spoons of butter and melt. Stir in the flour and cook, stirring, for 1 minute, until it is cooked.

4.Stir in the wine, tomatoes, stock, bay leaves, and hot pepper sauce. Reduce heat to medium-low and simmer for 16 minutes, periodically stirring.

5.Remove bay leaves. Using a spoon, push the shrimp mixture to one side of the pot. Pour the eggs into the opposite side, and begin to scramble. Stir the eggs into the shrimp mixture and again push to one side. Pour the rice into the pot and mix it in. Cover the pot, reduce the heat to low, and cook for 5 minutes longer to heat through.

6.Sprinkle with green onions when serving

Nutrition: Energy (calories): 1017 kcal Protein: 89.27 g Fat: 52.71 g Carbohydrates: 95.46 g Calcium, Ca322 mg Magnesium, Mg1400 mg Phosphorus, P3672 mg

Sweet & Smoky Pulled Chicken

Prep Time: 10 minutes

Cook Time: 20 minutes

Serve: 6

Ingredients:

- 750 g skinless and boneless chicken breasts (1.65 lb.) 400 ml unsweetened passata tomato (sauce) (13.5 fl oz) 100 ml apple cider vinegar (3.5 fl oz)
- 3 tbsp Erythritol or Swerve (30 g/ 1.1 oz)
- Optional: 1 tbsp of molasses (20 g/0.7 oz) - see note 1 tsp of sea salt above
- 1 black pepper tablespoon
- 1 TL garlic powder
- 1/4 tsp of Cayenne-pepper or 1 tbsp of smoked paprika to taste 3 tbsp of amino coconut (45 ml)
- 1/4 Cup of Virgin Olive Oil Extra (60 ml)
- Optional: 1 cup of sour cream, full-fat yogurt, or fresh cream for serving.

Instructions:

1.In a large bowl, place the chicken breasts and cover with the tomato passata. To that, add the ground or whole peppercorns, salt, black pepper, and garlic powder. Toss to combine and transfer to the crockpot. Toss again to coat and let it cook on low for 5 hours.

2. Cook the rice according to the direction of the box and move it to a big bowl. Add the sour cream, coconut cream, and Swerve. Whisk until combined.

3.Finely mince the fresh parsley. Mix the parsley and the smoked paprika with the rice. To serve, pile the rice onto the chicken and top with the sour cream or yogurt or creme fraiche.

Nutrition: Energy (calories): 2924 kcal Protein: 85.2 g Fat: 27.19 g Carbohydrates: 515.51 g Calcium, Ca578 mg Magnesium, Mg347 mg Phosphorus, P1475 mg

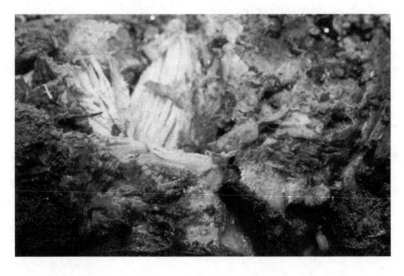

Garlic Crusted BBQ Baby Back Ribs

Prep Time: 15 minutes

Cook Time: 1-hour

Serve: 2

Ingredients:

- 11 and three-fourth rack baby back ribs 2 tablespoons extra-virgin olive oil Kosher salt and freshly ground pepper 6 clove garlic
- 12 sprig thyme
- 8 sage leaves with stems 2 sprig rosemary

Instructions:

1. To 350F, preheat the oven. With salt and pepper, season the ribs and poke them all over with a fork. Rub both sides with olive oil and put them over a baking sheet in a roasting rack package.

2.Sprinkle garlic over the meat, and place 4 sage leaves, 4 sage leaves with stems, and 4 rosemary leaves on top of the meat.

3.Bake the ribs for 30 minutes. Reduce the oven temperature to 310F and bake the ribs for 25 minutes. Place 4 more sage leaves, 4 sage leaves with stems, another 30 all the and brush

4.And 4 rosemary leaves on top of the meat. Bake for minutes.

5.Place 1 cup of barbecue sauce in a bowl. Scrape

6.Sauce from the roaster. Return the ribs to the pan the meat with the sauce. Bake for 15 additional minutes.

7.Scrape the sauce again from the roaster and spread it over the meat. More sauce.

8.Remove the meat from the oven and serve with

Nutrition: Energy (calories): 19863 kcal Protein: 1754.29 g Fat: 1401.07 g Carbohydrates: 82.05 g Calcium, Ca1903 mg Magnesium, Mg2170 mg Phosphorus, P12527 mg

Juicy Rosemary Pulled Pork

Prep Time: 10 minutes

Cook Time: 35 minutes

Serve: 4

Ingredients:

- 1 tbsp olive-oil 1 tsp sea salt
- 1/2 tsp ground black-pepper
- 4 boneless center-cut pork chops
- 6-8 cloves garlic, peeled and whole

Instructions:

1.Combine olive-oil, salt, and pepper in a small bowl. Rub into the pork chops. Refrigerate for 30 minutes.

2.Rub 2 cloves of garlic into the pork chops 2. Rub 2 cloves of garlic into the pork chops3. Preheat the grill. Grill pork chops 6-8 minutes on each side or until done.

3.Chop the remaining cloves of garlic. Add to a bowl with the rosemary, onion, and barbeque sauce. Mix to blend.

4.Preheat the oven to 325-degree F / 160 C.

5.Thinly slice the red-onion and place in a bowl. Add enough balsamic vinegar to cover and let marinate for 10 minutes.

6.In the same bowl, add the tomato halves. Sprinkle with garlic salt and olive oil. Stir to coat everything evenly.

7. In a baking dish, put the onions at the bottom of the dish. Place the pork chops on top and pour over any leftover marinade.

8.Cook covered for 30-35 minutes.

9.To make the sauce, place all the ingredients into a blender and blend until smooth.

10.Serve pork with sauce and lime wedges on the side.

Nutrition: Energy (calories): 265 kcal Protein: 39.52 g Fat: 10.02 g Carbohydrates: 1.98 g Calcium, Ca44 mg Magnesium, Mg48 mg Phosphorus, P400 mg

Slow-Cooked Chicken with Fire Roasted Tomatoes

Prep Time: 10 minutes

Cook Time: 3 hours and 10 minutes

Serve: 4

Ingredients:

- 1 1/2 lbs. boneless, skinless chicken breast
- 1 15oz can fire-roasted tomatoes (any variety- BUT make sure no extra added sugar)
- 2 T salt
- 2 T ground black pepper 2 T oil
- 2 T (one capful) sage
- 2 T (one capful) black pepper
- 2 T (one capful) onion and garlic

Instructions:

1.Add oil and chicken breasts to the slow cooker.

2.Pour a bottle of spices over the chicken and cover.

3.Cook on high for 3 hours.

4.Add fire-roasted tomatoes and cook for additional 10 minutes

5.Using a handheld blender or an upright blender, blend 6 tbsp of the liquid into the chicken.

6.Remove chicken and place on a plate.

7.Shred chicken into smaller pieces using two forks.

8.Serve over white or brown rice.

Nutrition: Energy (calories): 400 kcal Protein: 17.7 g Fat: 17.12 g Carbohydrates: 45.65 g Calcium, Ca131 mg Magnesium, Mg62 mg Phosphorus, P188 mg

Finger Licking BBQ Crock Pot Chicken

Prep Time: 10 minutes

Cook Time: 6 hours

Serve: 4

Ingredients:

- 1.5 lbs. – Boneless-Skinless-Chicken (thigh or breasts) 1 T – Stacey Hawkins Honey BBQ Seasoning
- 1 T – Stacey Hawkins Garlic & Spring Onion Seasoning 1 T – Phoenix Sunrise Seasoning

Instructions:

1.In a slow cooker, mix all of the seasonings.

2.Remove from the chicken any fat and skin and cut into equally-sized pieces.

3.Add chicken pieces to the seasonings in the slow cooker.

4.Drizzle 2T honey BBQ over the chicken pieces. Mix.

5.Cook for 5 ½ hours on a low setting.

6.Before serving, add one-fourth cup BBQ sauce to the chicken in the crockpot.

7.Mix thoroughly and cook for 6 minutes on high to let the BBQ sauce cook into the chicken.

Nutrition: Energy (calories): 400 kcal Protein: 17.7 g Fat: 17.12 g Carbohydrates: 45.65 g Calcium, Ca131 mg Magnesium, Mg62 mg Phosphorus, P188 mg

Big Mac in a Bowl

Prep Time: 10 minutes

Cook Time: 10 minutes

Serve: 4

Ingredients:

- 1 lb lean ground beef lean beef
- 1 tbsp of onion powder
- 1 Tbsp garlic Powder
- 2 or 3 dashes Worcestershire sauce
- 8 cups of roman lettuce
- 16 Pickle slices
- Fat cheddar reduced in 4 oz
- 8 tbsps of red, diced onion
- 2 diced Tomato Roma
- 8 Lite Thousand Island Dressing Spoons

Instructions:

1. Cook the ground beef in a nonstick skillet over medium-high heat. Drain any excess fat when the beef is brown and no longer pink in the middle. Add the ground onion, garlic powder, and Worcestershire sauce. Only set aside.

2. Attach the top of the lettuce with 2 cups of sliced romaine lettuce, pickles, tomatoes, onions, cheese, and ground beef.

3. Put 2 tbsps of Thousand Island dressing on top of the salad.

Nutrition: 1; Calories: 390; Sugar: 7.4g; Fat: 20.7; Carbohydrates: 15.4g;Fiber: 4.5g; Protein: 34.9g

Coconut Flour Chicken Nuggets

Ingredients:

- Thighs of 1 pound of skinless chicken
- 3/4 cup mayo
- 1/3 cup of flour with arrowroot
- 1/4 cup of flour for coconut
- 1/2 Tbsp powdered onion
- 1/2 Tbsp powdered garlic
- 1/4 tbsp of turmeric
- 1/2 tbsp of basil dried
- 1/2 tbsp oregano
- 1/4 tbsp Smoked Paprika
- 1/4 tsp of cayenne
- 1/4 tbsp of salt
- 1/8 tbsp of black pepper

Instructions:

1. Preheat to 450 ° F in the oven.

2. Put the parchment paper into a large baking sheet.

3. Combine the arrowroot starch, coconut meal, and spices in a dish.

4. Dip every piece of chicken into the mayo (or wash the eggs), then dip into the mixture of coconut flour. On the baking sheet, put the chicken and repeat for the remaining pieces of chicken.

5. Bake for twenty minutes at 450 ° F or until the juices from the chicken are clear.

Skinny Chicken Salad

Prep Time: 25 mins

Cook Time: 15 mins

Serve: 5

Ingredients:

- Boneless 1.5 lbs, skinless breast of chicken, fried ani finely shredded
- 2 chopped green onions
- 2 halved and chopped celery stalks
- 1/3 cup of congrats parsley
- ½ cup of paleo mayo
- 1/2 C Greek yogurt
- Juice from 1 lemon
- Salt and pepper

Instructions:

1. Chicken's generous season with salt and pepper and cook in a crockpot, instant pot, or cooked poach and no longer pink.

2. Move the cooked chicken to your stand mixer or cutting board to finely shred. Use the paddle connector and turn it to medium

speed while using a stand mixer and let it be shredded to your taste.

3. Place shredded chicken in a medium side mixing bowl to all other ingredients. Whisk to combine.

4. Serve over greens, on crostini's, etc., in a wrap, as a dip.

5. In an airtight jar in the fridge for 5 days.

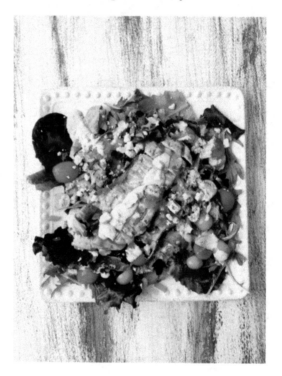

Chicken Marsala

Prep Time: 15 minutes

Cook Time: 20 minutes

Serve: 4

Ingredients:

- 1 1/4 cups of dry marsala wine
- 1 1/4 cups of unsalted chicken broth
- 2 (10 - 11 oz) pounded, boneless skinless chicken breasts Salt and freshly ground black pepper 1/3 cup of all purpose flour
- 2 Tbsp of unsalted butter
- 2 Tbsp of olive oil
- 8 oz. of sliced cremini mushrooms
- 3 1 Tbsp minced garlic cloves
- 1 tsp of minced fresh thyme
- 1 tsp of minced fresh oregano
- 1 1/2 tsp of cornstarch whisked with 1 Tbsp chicken broth (well combined)
- 1/3 cup of heavy cream
- 1 Tbsp of minced fresh parsley

Instructions:

1. To a medium saucepan, add marsala wine and chicken broth. Heat over medium-high-heat, bring to a boil, reduce to medium heat, and cook gently until it is reduced to 1 cup, about 15 min.

2. With salt and pepper, season the chicken on both sides.

3. Dredge in the flour mixture on either side.

4. In a 12-inch skillet over medium-high heat, melt 1 Tbsp of butter with 1 Tbsp of olive oil. Add pieces of chicken and let it sear until it is cooked through (165 in the center), turning around 10-12 minutes once halfway through.

5. Move your chicken to an oven. Tent on the foil.

6. Reduce burner to medium flame. Melt the remaining 1 tbsp of butter and 1 tbsp of olive oil, then add the mushrooms.

7. Stir in mushrooms, tossing just periodically (and growing the burner temp slightly as required to promote browning), until the mushrooms have shrunk and are golden brown, around 8 min. During last one minute of sautéing, add garlic.

8. Then pour in marsala reduction, thyme and oregano, remove the pan from fire.

9. Return to flame, bring to a simmer and scrape brown bits from the rim, then whisk in a mixture of cornstarch chicken broth. Delete to thickened.

10. Stir off heat in heavy cream, and season with salt and pepper to taste. Put the chicken breasts back in the pan, then spoon the sauce over the top.

11. Sprinkle and serve immediately with parsley.

Nutrition: Calories 448, Fat 24 g; Cholesterol 133 mg; Sodium 200 mg; Potassium 944 mg; Carbo. 11 g; Fiber 1 g; Sugar 3 g; Protein 33 g; Calcium 45 mg; Iron 2 mg

Turkey Meatloaf

Active Time: 30 min

Total Time: 1 1/2 hr

Ingredients:

- 1 1/2 cups of onion finely chopped
- 1 tbsp of minced garlic
- 1 tsp of olive oil
- 1 medium of carrot
- 3/4 pound trimmed and very finely chopped cremini mushrooms 1 tsp of salt
- 1/2 tsp of black pepper
- 1 1/2 tsps of Worcestershire sauce
- fresh parsley, finely chopped (1/3 cup)
- 1/4 cup of plus 1 tbsp ketchup
- Fine fresh bread crumbs (1 cup)
- 1/3 cup of milk
- 1 whole of a lightly beaten large egg
- 1 large lightly beaten egg white
- 1 1/4 pound of ground turkey Accompaniment: roasted red pepper tomato sauce

Instructions:

1. Preheat the oven to 204.444°C.

2. In a 11-inch nonstick skillet, cook the onion and garlic in oil over moderate heat, stirring, until the onion is tender, around 2 minutes. Add carrot and cook, stirring for about 3 minutes, until softened. Add mushrooms, 1/2 tsp of salt, and 1/4 tsp of pepper and cook, occasionally stirring, until liquid mushrooms are evaporated and very tender, 10 to 15 minutes. Stir in Worcestershire sauce, parsley, and ketchup for 3 tsps, then switch vegetables to a large bowl and cool down.

3. In a small cup, mix together the bread crumbs and milk and let stand for 5 minutes. Stir in the white egg and egg, and add to the vegetables. Apply the turkey and remaining 1/2 tsp salt and 1/4 tsp pepper to the mixture of vegetables and blend well with hands. (The mixture was going to be very humid.)

4. In a lightly oiled 13- by 9- by 2-inch metal baking pan, shape a 9- by 5-inch oval loaf and brush meatloaf evenly with the remaining 2 tablespoons ketchup. Bake in the center of the oven until 170 ° F, 50 to 55 minutes of thermometer inserted into meatloaf registers.

5. Let meatloaf to stand five minutes before serving.

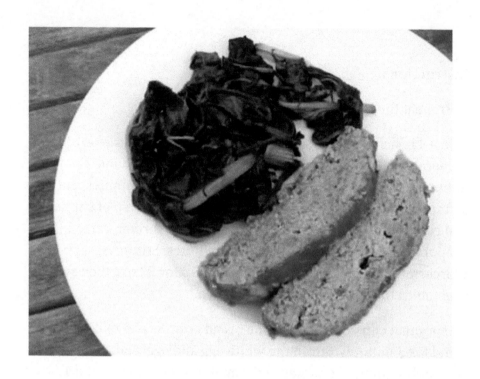

Chicken Piccata

Ingredients:

- ½ cup of reduced-sodium chicken broth 2 tsp of cornstarch
- 2 (8 ounces) skinless, boneless chicken breast halved ¼ cup of all-purpose flour ½ tsp of kosher salt
- black pepper freshly ground (1 tsp)
- 4 tsp of olive oil
- 4 lemon slices
- 2 tsp of butter
- 3 large minced cloves garlic
- ¼ cup of dry white wine
- 2 tbsp of lemon juice
- 1 ½ tbsp. of drained capers
- 1 ½ tsp of snipped fresh thyme

Instructions:

1. Stir together the broth and the cornstarch in a small bowl; set aside. Flatten the chicken between two sheets of plastic wrap until 1/2 inch thick using the flat side of a meat mallet. Stir together rice, salt, and pepper in a shallow dish. Sprinkle the chicken into a mixture of flour, turning to cover.

2. Hot oil over medium-high heat in a 12-inch nonstick skillet. Add chicken; cook 8 to 9 minutes, turning once. Withdraw from the skillet; keep warm. Add lemon slices to skillet if necessary. Cook for 30 to 60 seconds or, turning once, until brown. Take off the skillet.

3. For the sauce, melt butter over medium in skillet. Add the garlic for 30 seconds, cook and stir. Put the wine in carefully. Cook for one to two minutes or until slightly thick, stirring up crusty brown bits to scrape. Stir in a mixture of cornstarch. Take to boil; minimize heat. Simmer for 1 minute, or until dense. Incorporate lemon juice, capers, and thyme.

4. Drizzle the chicken with the sauce and top with the slices of lemon and extra thyme.

Nutrition: 249 calories; total fat 9.6g 15% DV; saturated fat 2.5g; cholesterol 88mg 29% DV; sodium 354mg 14% DV; potassium 461mg 13% DV; carbohydrates 9.7g 3% DV; fiber 0.6g 2% DV; sugarg; protein 27.2g 54% DV; exchange other carbs 1; vitamin a iu 274IU; vitamin c 7mg; folate 39mcg; calcium 23mg; iron 1mg; magnesium 39mg.

Chicken, Bell Pepper & Carrot Curry

Prep Time: 15 minutes

Cook Time: 12 minutes

Serve: 4

Ingredients:

- 1 (14-ounce) can unsweetened coconut milk
- 2 tablespoons Thai red curry paste
- 1 pound of boneless-chicken breast cut into thin pieces
- 1 cup carrots, peeled and sliced
- 1½ cups green bell pepper, seeded and cubed
- ½ cup onion, sliced ¼ cup chicken broth
- 2 tablespoon fish sauce
- 1 tablespoon fresh lime juice
- 12 fresh basil leaves, chopped
- Salt and ground black pepper, as required.

Instructions:

1. Add the oil to Instant Pot and select "Sauté." Then add half of coconut milk and curry paste and cook for about 1-2 minutes.

2. Press "Cancel" and stir in remaining coconut milk, chicken, carrot, bell pepper, onion, and broth.

3. Secure the lid and switch to the location of the "Seal".

4. Cook on "Manual" with "High Pressure" for about 5 minutes.

5. Press "Cancel" and carefully do a "Quick" release.

6. Remove the lid and select "Sauté".

7. For the rest of the ingredients, stir in and cook for 4-5 minutes or so.

8. Stir in the salt and black pepper and press "Cancel".

Nutrition: Calories: 282 | fat: 24.0g | protein: 10.1g | carbs: 6.9g | net carbs: 2.8g | fiber: 4.1g

Chicken Chili

Prep Time: 15 minutes

Cook Time: 20 minutes

Serve: 4

Ingredients:

- 3 (5-ounce) chicken breasts
- 1 carrot, peeled and chopped
- 1 celery stalk, chopped
- 1 medium yellow onion, chopped
- 2 garlic cloves, chopped
- 1 teaspoon dried oregano
- 1 teaspoon ground cumin
- Salt and ground black pepper, as required
- ½ cup unsweetened coconut milk
- 1 cup chicken broth

Instructions:

1.Ad all the ingredients to the Instant Pot pot and mix to blend.

2.Secure the lid and switch to the location of the "Seal".

3.Select "Poultry" and just use the default time of 20 minutes.

4.Press "Cancel" and do a "Natural" release.

5.Remove the lid and, with a slotted spoon, transfer the chicken breasts into a bowl.

6.With 2 forks, shred chicken breasts and then return into the pot.

Nutrition: Calories: 306 | fat: 15.6g | protein: 33.4g | carbs: 7.1g | net carbs: 5.2g | fiber: 1.9g

Beef and Kale Casserole

Prep Time: 15 minutes

Cook Time: 29 minutes

Serve: 4

Ingredients:

- 2 tablespoons olive oil
- 2 cups fresh kale, trimmed and chopped
- 1 1/3 cups scallion, sliced
- 8 egg, beaten
- 1½ cups cooked beef, shredded
- Salt and ground black pepper, as required

Instructions:

1. In the Instant Pot, add oil and pick "Sauté". Then add the kale and scallion and cook for about 3-4 minutes.

2. Press "Cancel" and transfer the kale mixture into a bowl.

3. Add eggs and beef and mix well.

4. Move the mixture into a baking dish that is lightly greased.

5. Arrange a steamer trivet in the lower part of the Instant Pot and pour 1½ cups of water.

6. Place the baking dish on top of the trivet.

7. Secure the lid and turn to the "Seal" position.

8. Cook on "Manual" with "High Pressure" for about 25 minutes.

9. Press "Cancel" and carefully do a "Quick" release.

10. Remove the lid and serve immediately.

Nutrition: calories: 345 | fat: 20.2g | protein: 34.2g | carbs: 6.6g | net carbs: 5.2g | fiber: 1.4g

Beef and Mushroom Soup

Prep Time: 15 minutes

Cook Time: 15 minutes

Serve: 4

Ingredients:

- 2 teaspoons olive oil
- 1 pound sirloin steak, trimmed and cubed
- 1 small carrot, peeled and chopped
- 1 bell pepper, seeded and chopped
- 1 celery stalk, chopped
- 1 onion, chopped
- 8 ounces fresh mushrooms, sliced
- 2 cups beef broth
- 1½ cups water
- 1 cup tomatoes, crushed
- 1½ tablespoons fresh oregano chopped 1 bay leaf
- 2 teaspoon garlic powder
- Salt and ground black pepper, as required

Instructions:

1. Add the oil in an Instant Pot Mini and select "Sauté". Now, add the steak and cook for about 4-5 minutes or until browned.

2. Add the carrots, bell pepper, celery, and onion and cook for about 2-3 minutes.

3. Attach the mushrooms, then cook for 4-5 minutes or so.

4. Push and stir in the remaining ingredients with "Cancel".

5. Secure the lid and turn to the "Seal" position.

6. Select "Soup" and just use the default time of 15 minutes.

7. Press "Cancel" and do a "Quick" release.

8. Remove the lid and serve hot.

Nutrition: Calories: 298 | fat: 10.6g | protein: 39.9g | carbs: 10g | net carbs: 6.7g | fiber: 3.3g

Salmon with cucumbers, tomatoes, and dill salad

Total time: 30 minutes

Serve: 4

Ingredients:

- 1-pint cherry tomatoes (cut in half)
- 4 cups cucumber (sliced)
- ¼ cup cider vinegar
- ¼ cup dill (chopped)
- ¼ tsp. salt
- ¼ tsp. black pepper
- 1½ lbs. salmon (skinless)
- 1 tbsp. Za'atar
- 4 lemon wedges

Instructions:

1.Preheat the oven to 350°F.

2.In the meantime, prepare the salad. Take a bowl and put the sliced cucumbers, the cherry tomatoes, the cider vinegar, and the chopped dill. Toss everything until thoroughly combined.

3.Now, take the salmon and season it with Za'atar on both sides, and place them on a tray. Roast the salmon until it reaches the temperature of 145°F.

4.When ready, serve the salmon with the salad and lemon wedges.

Salmon burgers with cucumber salad

Total time: 25 minutes

Serve: 2

Ingredients:

- 1 egg (slightly beaten)
- 1½ tbsp. light mayo
- ½ tsp. lemon juice
- 1 tbsp. onion (diced)
- ¼ tsp. dried parsley
- dash of pepper
- 1,5 oz. salmon (skinless, boneless, and can drain)
- 1 packet of multigrain crackers (crushed)
- cooking spray
- 1,5 oz. low-fat Greek yogurt
- 2 tbsp. apple cider vinegar
- 1 tbsp. dill
- dash of salt
- 3 cups cucumber (peeled and thinly sliced)

Instructions:

1.Take a bowl and whisk together the egg, mayo, lemon juice, onion, parsley, and pepper. Gently fold in salmon and crushed crackers. Break the mixture, then form it into two patties. Cook on a lightly greased pan over medium-high heat until golden brown on both sides (about 5 minutes per side).

2.Meanwhile, whisk together the Greek yogurt, apple cider vinegar, dill, salt, and pepper. Pour over cucumber slices, and stir to mix in Chill until ready to serve.

Roasted red pepper sauce scallops and zucchini noodles

Total time: 30 minutes

Serve: 2

Ingredients:

- 6 oz. jarred roasted red peppers (drained)
- ½ cup unsweetened almond or cashew milk
- 2 oz. avocado
- 2 tsp. lemon juice
- 1 clove garlic
- ¼ tsp. red pepper (crushed)
- ¼ tsp + 1/8 tsp salt
- 2 small zucchini (cut into spaghetti-like strands)
- ½ tbsp. butter
- 1 lbs. raw scallops

Instructions:

1. Place the roasted red peppers, milk, avocado, lemon juice, garlic, crushed red pepper and 1/4 tsp. in a blender.

2.Heat roasted red-pepper sauce in a pan over medium heat, occasionally stirring, for about 3-5 minutes. Then, add zucchini

49

noodles, stir to incorporate, and continue cooking until cooked to your liking (about 3-5 minutes).

3. Meanwhile, in a broad skillet over medium-high heat, melt-butter. With the remaining salt, season the scallops. Cook the scallops until golden brown on each side and translucent in the centre (about 1-2 minutes per side).

4.Serve zucchini noodles with scallops on top.

Stir-fried winter melon with shrimp

Total Time: 30 minutes

Serve: 4

Ingredients:

- 4 tsp. olive oil
- 1 tbsp. ginger root (peeled and minced)
- 1 scallion (trimmed and minced)
- 30 oz. raw shrimp (peeled and deveined)
- ½ tsp. salt (divided)
- 4 tsp. canola oil
- 6 cups winter melon (trimmed and sliced)
- ½ cup water
- ½ tsp. black pepper
- 2 tsp. fresh chili paste
- ¼ cup coriander (chopped)

Instructions:

1.Heat the mustard oil in a non-stick wok or skillet and gently cook the ginger and scallion until fragrant.

2.Add the shrimp to the wok and continue to stir fry until pink. Add half the salt.

51

3.Once the shrimp are cookeed, remove them from the wok or skillet and set aside.

4.In the same wook or skillet, heat the canola oil. Add the sliced winter melon, and stir-fry over medium heat until they become tender (about 5-8 minutes). Add the water as needed and cover with a lid. Adjust seasoning with the remaining salt and add the pepper.

5.Return the shrimp into the same wok or skillet, heat through. Add the chili paste and green coriander and serve warm.

Roasted lemon pepper salmon and garlic Parmesan asparagus

Total time: 35 minutes

Serve: 4

Ingredients:

- 1½ lbs. salmon (skin on)
- 2½ tbsp. olive oil
- 1 tsp. lemon zest
- 1 tbsp. fresh lemon juice
- 4 cloves garlic (minced)
- 1 tsp. Dijon mustard
- ¾ tsp. onion powder
- ½ tsp. each salt and black pepper (plus more for asparagus)
- ½ lemon (thinly sliced)
- 1½ – 2 lbs. asparagus (ends trimmed)
- ½ cup parmesan (finely shredded)

Instructions:

1.Preheat oven to 400°F. Place salmon in the ceenter of the pan. In a mixing bowl, whisk together 1½ tbsp of olive oil, the lemon zest, lemon juice, 2 cloves of garlic, Dijon mustard, and onion powder.

Brush evenly over the top of the salmon, and then sprinkle ½ tsp. of salt and black pepper. Arrange lemon slices on top.

2.Toss asparagus with 1 tbsp. Of olive oil, 2 cloves of garlic and season with salt, then place around salmon. Bake in a preheated oven (about 10 minutes).

3.Remove from oven, toss asparagus, then sprinkle asparagus with Parmesan. After sprinkling the Parmesan, put it into the oven and bake it until salmon has cooked through (about 5 – 10 minutes). Cut salmon into portions and serve it warm.

Avocado lime shrimp salad

Total time: 15 minutes

Serve: 2

Ingredients:

- 14 oz. jumbo cooked shrimp (peeled and deveined, chopped)
- 1½ cup tomato (diced)
- 4½ oz. avocado (diced)
- ¼ cup jalapeño (seeds removed, finely diced)
- ¼ cup green onion (chopped)
- 2 tbsp. lime juice
- 1 tsp. olive oil
- 1 tbsp. coriander (chopped)
- 1/8 tsp. salt
- ¼ tsp. black pepper

Instructions:

1.Take a bowl and combine green onion, lime juice, olive oil, a pinch of salt, and pepper. Let them marinate to soften the onion (at least 5 minutes).

2.In a bowl, mix in chopped shrimp, avocado, tomato, jalapeño. Combine all the ingredients, add coriander, and gently toss. Adjust salt and pepper to taste.

Steamed Seafood Pot

Total Time: 1 hour 15 minutes

Serve: 4

Ingredients:

- 14 oz. winter melon (peeled, seeded, and thinly sliced)
- 7 oz. Oriental radish (peeled and thinly sliced)
- 17 oz. Chinese cabbage (wash, drain, and sliced)
- 21 oz. firm tofu (drain and sliced)
- 11 oz. fresh prawns with shells (washed and drained)
- 32 oz. fresh clams with shell (cover with water and 1 tsp. of salt for 1 hour to remove the sands, washed and drained)
- 4 blue crabs with shells (about 35 oz., washed and drained)
- 1 cup water
- ½ cup fresh coriander
- 1 scallion (trimmed and chopped)
- 2 fresh red hot chilies (cut into half and remove seeds)
- 2 tbsp. soy sauce
- 4 tsp. sesame oil

Instructions:

1.Layer the winter melon, Oriental radish, and cabbage at the bottom of the pot.

2.Layer tofu slices on top of the vegetables.

3.Spread prawns, clams, and crabs on top.

4. Place the water on the side of the bowl. Cover the lid and cook until all the ingredients are well cooked (about 15 minutes).

5.Garnish with coriander and scallions. Serve with chili, soy sauce, and sesame oil.

Avocado lime tuna salad

Total time: 15 minutes

Serve: 4

Ingredients:

- 3 cans of tuna water (drained)
- 1 cup cucumber (quartered and sliced)
- 1 avocado (seeded, peeled, and diced)
- 2 tbsp. onion (thinly sliced)
- ¼ cup coriander (chopped)
- 2 tbsp. lime juice
- ¼ cup olive oil
- ½ tsp. chili powder
- ¼ tsp. cumin
- salt and black pepper to taste

Instructions:

1.take a bowl and place the tuna, cucumber, avocado, onion, and coriander.

2.In another bowl, whisk together the lime juice, olive oil, chili powder, cumin, salt, and black pepper.

3.Over the tuna mixture, add the dressing; toss gently to cover.

Low-carb lobster roll

Total Time: 15 minutes

Serve: 2

Ingredients:

- 2 small heads of romaine lettuce
- 1 tbsp. butter (melted)
- 1/3 cup Greek yogurt (low-fat)
- 2 tbsp. mayonnaise
- 1 small stalk celery (finely diced)
- 2 tsp. lemon juice
- 1 tbsp. chives (chopped)
- ¼ tsp. paprika
- ¼ tsp. salt
- ¼ tsp. pepper
- 12 oz. cooked lobster meat

Instructions:

1.Preheat grill.

2.Slice romaine hearts in half lengthwise. Remove one or two of the inner leaves from each half to create a boat-like shape for the lobster filling. Lightly coat the inner parts and edges of each "boat" with butter, and grill cut-side-down to get a slight char and bring out the lettuce's flavors (about 2-3 minutes).

3.Take a bowl and mix the remaining ingredients except for the lobster meat. Once ingredients are well mixed, fold in the lobster meat until completely coated.

4.Arrange the lobster mixture evenly among the boats.

Noodle soup

Total Time: 45 minutes

Serve: 4

Ingredients:

- 8 oz. Celtuce ("spiralized" into noodle-like strands)
- 4 cups of water
- 3 oz. lemongrass sticks (mashed and cut into 2 inches long)
- 4 shallots (peeled and sliced)
- 0.3 oz. Thai lime leaves
- 2.4 oz. blue ginger (sliced)
- 2 pieces fresh red hot chili (cut in half, seeds and membranes removed)
- 2 medium tomatoes (cut each tomato into 6 wedges)
- 14 oz. firm tofu (cut into ½inch x ½inch cubes)
- 2 cups oyster mushrooms (sliced)
- 10 oz. frozen shrimps (defrost, washed, and drained)
- 10 oz. frozen scallops (defrost, washed, and drained)
- 2 tbsp. fish sauce
- ½ cup coconut milk
- 2 tbsp. lime juice
- ½ cup fresh coriander (slightly chopped)

Instructions:

1.Take a pot, pour waater into it, and bring it to a boil. Add the Celtuce "noodles" and cook for 2 minutes. Drain the noodlees, put them in a bowl on the side.

2.Take a pot, pour water into it. When the water is boiling, add lemongrass, shallots, Thai lime leaves, blue ginger, chili, tomatoes, tofu, and mushrooms. Cook for about 3 minutes.

3.Add shrimp and scalloops and cook for 3,3 minutes.

4.Turn off the heat, add fish sauce, coconut milk, and lime juice. Stir to combine well.

5.Carefully remove the lemongrass sticks, shallot slices, Thai lime leaves, and blue ginger with a slotted spoon.

6.Pour the soup over the Celtuce "noodles." Garnish with coriander leaves.

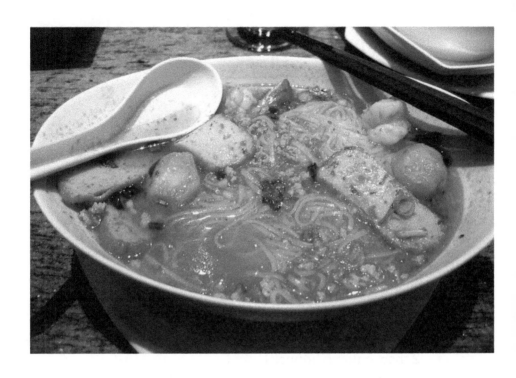

Steamed white fish street tacos

Total Time: 20 minutes

Serve: 2

Ingredients:

- 16 oz. raw cod fillets
- ½ tsp. garlic powder
- ½ tsp. salt, divided
- ½ cup tomato (diced)
- 2 tbsp. onion (chopped)
- ½ jalapeño pepper (seeds and membranes removed, chopped)
- 2 tbsp. cilantro (chopped)
- 1 tbsp. lime juice
- 6 large romaine lettuce leaves
- 1 avocado (about 6 oz., sliced)

Instructions:

1.Season cod with garlic powder and ¼ tsp. of salt. Steam fish until cooked through (about 5-10 minutes). Flake the fish, using a fork, removing any bones.

2.Meanwhile, prepare pico de gallo. Take a bowl and combine tomato, onion, jalapeño pepper, cilantro, lime juice, and the remaining salt.

3.To prepare tacos: Top each romaine lettuce leaf with fish, avocado, and pico de gallo.

Stir-fry shrimps with champignon mushroom and broccoli

Total time: 25 minutes

Serve: 4

Ingredients:

- 1 lb. shrimps
- 2 garlic cloves
- 1 onion (chopped)
- 1 crown broccoli (chopped)
- ¼ lb. champignon mushroom
- 1 tbsp. + 2 tsp. corn starch
- 2 tbsp. soy sauce
- 1 tsp. rice vinegar
- ½ tbsp. brown sugar
- ½ cup chicken broth
- 2 tbsp. canola oil
- ½ tbsp. lemon juice

Instructions:

1.Take the shrimps and mix them with 1 tbsp. Of corn starch, then ass salt and pepper to taste.

2.Take the soy sauce and mix it with vinegar, brown sugar, chicken broth, and 2 tsp. Corn starch.

3.Now take the wok and put it over medium-high heat. Add 1 tbsp. Of canola oil, heat it, and then add the shrimps to it. Cooked the shrimps until they will get a golden color. Then remove the shrimps from the pan and set aside.

4.Once you removed the shrimps from the pan, put it over medium-high heat, and add the remaining canola oil. Now, add the garlic cloves and then the chopped onions with a dash of salt. Cooked the onions until they become soft (about 2 minutes).

5.Add broccoli and season them with a bit of salt. Stir-fry for about 2 minutes, add sliced champignon mushrooms, and season them with a salt dash.

6.Now, add the shrimps back in. Push all the ingredients to the pan's side to form a circle in the middle. Then, put the sauce mixture into the pan's center (in case the corn starch has sunk to the bottom, stir it).

7.Cook until shrimps are ready. Then, remove the pan from heat and add1/2 tbs. of lemon juice. Add salt and pepper to taste.

Steamed stuffed mushrooms (with pork)

Total Time: 30 minutes

Serve: 2

Ingredients:

- 6 oz. raw pork tenderloin (minced into bite-sized pieces)
- 7 oz. cooked shrimp (peeled, deveined, and minced into bite-sized pieces)
- 7 oz. fresh white mushrooms (stems removed)
- 2 tbsp. soy sauce
- 1 tbsp. rice wine vinegar
- 2 tsp. sesame oil
- ¼ tsp. black pepper
- 1 spring onion (trimmed and minced)
- ½ tsp. chili oil

Instructions:

1. Combine minced pork and shrimp with soy sauce, vinegar, oil, and pepper. Marinate for at least one hour. Drain liquid when finished.

2. When ready to serve, stuff each mushroom cap with the pork and shrimp mixture and place on a steamer plate (if needed, put

any extra meat and shrimp alongside the mushrooms on the plate). Steam on the stovetop until the meat and shrimp are fully cooked (about 15 minutes).

3.Garnish with spring onions and chili oil.

Sheet pan shrimp scampi

Total Time: 15 minutes

Serve: 2

Ingredients:

- 12 oz. zucchini (ends removed)
- 16 oz. raw shrimp (peeled and deveined)
- 2 tbsp. grated Parmesan cheese
- Juice of half a lemon
- 1 tbsp. butter (unsalted, melted)
- 2 tsp. olive oil
- 1 clove garlic (minced)
- ¼ tsp. salt

Instructions:

1.Preheat oven to 400°F.

2.Using a vegetable peeler, cut zucchini into thin strips.

3.Then, take a re-sealable plastic bag and combine zucchini strips and the remaining ingredients. Seal the bag and toss it to evenly coat zucchini and shrimp.

4.Distribute the mixture in an even layer onto a foil-lined baking sheet. Bake until shrimp are cooked through (about 8 minutes).

Sambal Kang Kong with bay scallops

Total Time: 30 minutes

Serve: 4

Ingredients:

- 6 scallions (trimmed and chopped)
- 2 garlic cloves (chopped)
- 1 tbsp. lemongrass (minced)
- 2 tsp. ginger root (peeled and minced)
- 1 tbsp. chili paste
- 2 fresh Thai bird chilies (seeds and membranes removed)
- 1 tbsp. shrimp paste
- 4 tsp. lime juice
- 2 tbsp. + 2 tsp. canola oil
- 25 oz. bay scallops
- 25 oz. water spinach
- 1 tbsp. fish sauce

Instructions:

1.Combine the scallions, garlic, lemongrass, ginger, chili paste, Thai bird chilies, shrimp paste, and lime juice in a blender and puree fine paste, adding water as needed to facilitate blending.

Alternatively, you can use a pestle and a mortar. Set the paste aside when done.

2.Heat 2 tsp. Oil in a wok or pan-and add the scallops, and stir-fry until almost cooked through (about 3-5 minutes). Remove from the wok, put them on the side, and keep warm.

3.Heat the remaining 2 tbsp. Of oil in the same wook or skillet and cook the spice paste over moderate heat until almost dry (about 5 to 6 minutes).

4.Add the water spinach, fish sauce, and cook quickly until the spinach is wilted (about 3-5 minutes).

5.Arrange the water spinach on a platter and top with the scallops.

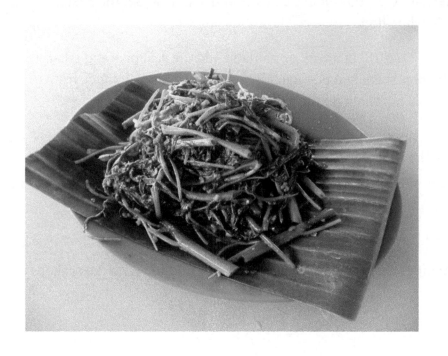

74

Crab and asparagus frittata

Total Time: 30 minutes

Serve: 4

Ingredients:

- 2½ tbsp. extra virgin olive oil
- 2 lbs. asparagus
- 1 tsp. salt
- ½ tsp black pepper
- 2 tsp sweet paprika
- 1 lb. lump crabmeat
- 1 tbsp. chives (finely cut)
- ¼ cup basil (chopped)
- 4 cups liquid egg substitute

Instructions:

1.Remove the ends of the asparaagus and cut it into small pieces.

2.Pre-heat an oven to 375°F.

3.In a 12-inch to 14-inch tray, heat the olive oil and gently sweat the asparagus until tender; then, season them with salt, pepper, and paprika.

4.In a bowl, add the chives, basil, and crab meat. Pour in the eggbeaters and gently mix until combined.

5.Carefully pour the crab and egg mixture into the tray with the cooked asparagus, and gently stir to combine. Cook over low to meedium heat until the egg beaters start bubbling.

6.Placee the tray in the oven and bake until the egg beaters are fully cooked and golden brown (about 15-20 minutes). Serve warm.

Shrimp and cauliflower grits

Total Time: 20 minutes

Serve: 2

Ingredients:

- 1 lb. shrimp (raw and peeled)
- ½ tbsp. Cajun seasoning
- cooking spray
- 1 tbsp. lemon juice
- ¼ cup chicken broth
- 1 tbsp. butter
- 2 ½ cups cauliflower (finely riced)
- ½ almond or cashew milk (unsweetened)
- ¼ cup sour cream
- ¼ tsp. salt
- 1/3 cup cheddar cheese (low-fat)
- ¼ cup scallions (thinly sliced)

Instructions:

1.In a big, re-sealable plastic bag, placed the shrimp and Cajun seasoning. Close the bag and toss in the seasoning to coat the shrimp evenly.

2. Use cooking spray to spray a pan and heat over medium heat. Cook the shrimp (about 2,3-3,3 minutes on each side) until yellow. Then add the chicken broth and lemon juice, boil for 1 minute, and then place it on the side.

3. Heat the butteer in a separate pan over medium heat. Connect the cauliflower 'riced' and cook (about 5 minutes). Add the milk and salt, then cook for an extra 5 minutes.

4.Remove pan from heat, and stir in sour cream and cheese until melted.

5.Serve shrimps atop cauliflower grits, and top with scallions.

Zucchini sheet with shrimp and scampi

Total Time: 15minutes

Serve: 2

Ingredients:

- 3 small zucchini (ends removed)
- 1 lb. raw shrimp (peeled and deveined)
- 2 tbsp. grated Parmesan cheese
- juice of half a lemon
- 1 tbsp. butter (unsalted, melted)
- 2 tsp. olive oil
- 1 clove garlic (minced)
- ¼ tsp. salt

Instructions:

1.Preheat oven to 400 °F.

2.Peel the zucchini into thin-ribbons using a vegetable peeler.

3. Combine the zucchini ribbons and residual ingredients in a large resealable plastic container. Seal the bag and toss well to mix all the ingredients together.

4. Spread the mixture onto a tray in an even layer and place it in the oven. Bake until the shrimp is cooked (about 8 minutes).

Crab zucchini sushi rolls

Total Time: 15minutes

Serve: 4

Ingredients:

- 3 cups lump crab meat
- 1 cup of Greek yogurt (low-fat)
- 2 tbsp. Sriracha sauce
- 1 medium avocado (peeled and sliced)
- 4 medium zucchini (remove ends)
- 1 small cucumber (chopped into matchstick-sized pieces)
- ¼ cup of soy sauce

Instructions:

1.Take a bowl and combine the crab meat with the Greek yogurt and the Sriracha sauce.

2.Take the zucchini and use a vegetable peeler or mandolin slicer to peel them into long, thin strips (8 per zucchini).

3.Lay the zucchini strips flat vertically and spread a spoonful (about 1-2 tbsp. of mixture per strip) of crab mixture on each one.

On each strip, place a few matchsticks of cucumber and a slice of avocado horizontally.

4. Roll up the strips of zucchini, secure them with toothpicks, and serve.

Oyster omelet

Total Time: 30 minutes

Serve: 4

Ingredients:

- 10 eggs
- 10 oz. oysters (chopped)
- 1 tbsp. soy sauce
- 1 tsp. canola oil
- 3 garlic cloves (minced)
- 1 tbsp. ginger root (peeled and minced)
- 1 scallion (trimmed and diced)
- 2 medium red bell peppers (8 oz., deseeded, deveined, and diced)
- 8 cups baby spinach

Instructions:

1.Take a bowl and combine eggs, oysters, light soy sauce, and beat with a fork. Put it on the side.

2.Take a pan and heat oil over medium-high heat. Add garlic, ginger, scallions, and red bell peppers. Sauté until aromatic.

3.Pour the beeaten egg mixture into the pan and gently push the cooked portion from the center's edges.

4.Keep cooking, tilting the pan, and moving the cooked portions gently as required.

5.When the top surface of eggs is set, and no visible liquid egg remains, place spinach on top and cover with a lid to wilt. The omelet is folded in half and moved to a tray. Serve hot or room temperature.

Spicy crab stuffed avocado

Total time: 10 minutes

Serve: 1

Ingredients:

- 2 tbsp. light mayo
- 2 tsp. sriracha (plus more for drizzling)
- 1 tsp. chives (chopped)
- 4 oz. lump crab meat
- ¼ cup cucumber (peeled and diced)
- 1 small avocado (4 oz., pitted and peeled)
- ½ tsp. furikake
- 2 tsp. soy sauce

Instructions:

1.Take a bowl and combine mayo, sriracha, and chives.

2.Add crab meat and cucumber and gently toss.

3.Cut the avocado open, remove the pit, peel the skin, or spoon the avocado.

4.Fill the avocado halves with crab salad in the same way.

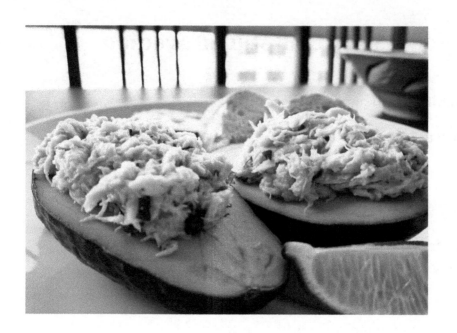

Blackened shrimp lettuce wraps

Total time: 20 minutes

Serve: 4

Ingredients:

- 2 lb. raw shrimp, peeled and deveined
- 1 tbsp. blackened seasoning
- 4 tsp. olive oil (divided)
- 1 cup of Greek yogurt (low-fat)
- 6 oz. avocado
- 2 tbsp. lime juice (divided)
- 1 ½ cups diced tomato
- ¼ cup green bell pepper (diced)
- ¼ cup onion (chopped)
- ¼ cup coriander (chopped)
- 1 jalapeño (chopped and deseeded)
- 12 large romaine lettuce leaves

Instructions:

1.In a re-sealable plastic bag, put the shrimp and blackened seasoning (you will need to split the shrimp into two batches). Shake the contents of the sack to uniformly disperse the seasoning.

2.Heat two teaspoons. In a saucepan, add olive oil and half the shrimp in a single layer. Cook until the shrimp is pink and fried. (approximately 2 to 3 minutes per side). Repeat with remaining shrimp and olive oil.

3.For the avocado salsa: combine Greek yogurt, avocado, and one tbsp. In a food proceessor, add lime juice and blend until smooth.

4.For the tomato salsa: take a bowl and stir the tomatoes, green bell pepper, onion, coriander, jalapeño, and remaining tbsp of lime juice.

5.Prepare lettuce wraps by dividing the shrimp, avocado salsa, and tomato salsa evenly among the lettuce leaves.

Beef & Veggies Stew

Prep Time: 15 minutes

Cook Time: 45 minutes

Serve: 4

Ingredients:

- 1¼ pounds beef stew meat, cubed
- 2 small zucchinis, chopped
- ½ pound small broccoli florets
- 2 garlic cloves, minced
- ½ cup chicken broth
- 1 tablespoon curry powder
- 1 teaspoon ground cumin
- Salt and ground black pepper, as required 7 ounces unsweetened coconut milk 2 tablespoons fresh cilantro, chopped.

Instructions:

1. In the pot of Instant Pot, place all ingredients except coconut milk and cilantro and stir to combine.

2. Secure the lid and turn to the "Seal" position.

3. For about 45 minutes cook on "Manual" with "High Pressure".

4. Click "Cancel" and perform a "Natural" release carefully for about 10 minutes. Then do a "Quick" release.

5. Stir in the coconut milk and remove the cap.

6. Serve immediately with the garnishing of cilantro.

Nutrition: Calories: 389 | fat: 17.9g | protein: 46.7g | carbs: 10g | net carbs: 7g | fiber: 3g

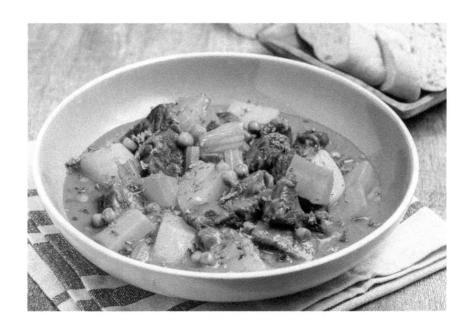

Beef & Carrot Chili

Prep Time: 15 minutes

Cook Time: 40 minutes

Serve: 4

Ingredients:

- 1 tablespoon olive oil
- 1 pound ground beef
- ½ green bell pepper, seeded and chopped
- 1 small onion, chopped
- 1 medium carrot, peeled and chopped
- 2 tomatoes, chopped finely
- 1 jalapeño pepper, chopped
- Salt and ground black-pepper, as required 1 tablespoon fresh parsley, chopped
- 1 tablespoon Worcestershire sauce
- 4 teaspoons red chili powder
- 1 teaspoon paprika
- 1 teaspoon ground cumin

Instructions:

1. Add the Instant Pot oil and pick 'Sauté.' Then add the beef and cook for

approximately 5 minutes or until fully browned.

2. Push and stir in the remaining ingredients with 'Cancel'.

3. Secure the lid and turn to the "Seal" position.

4. Choose 'Soup' and use the default time of 35 minutes only.

5. Press "Cancel" and do a "Natural" release.

6. Remove the lid and serve hot.

Nutrition: Calories: 287 | fat: 11.4g | protein: 36g | carbs: 9g | net carbs: 6g | fiber: 3g

Beef & Carrot Curry

Prep Time: 15 minutes

Cook Time: 33 minutes

Serve: 4

Ingredients:

- 2 tablespoons olive oil
- 1¼ pounds of stew meat with beef, cut into 1-inch sections Salt and ground black pepper, as required 1 cup onion, chopped
- 1 tablespoon fresh ginger, minced
- 2 teaspoons garlic, minced
- 1 jalapeño pepper, chopped finely
- 1 tablespoon curry powder
- 1 teaspoon red chili powder
- 1 teaspoon ground cumin
- 2 cups beef broth
- 1½ cups carrots, peeled and cut into 1-inch pieces 1 cup unsweetened coconut milk
- ¼ cup fresh cilantro, chopped

Instructions:

1. Add the oil in an Instant Pot Mini and select "Sauté". Now, add the beef, salt, and black pepper and cook for about 4-5 minutes or until browned completely.

2. Move the beef into a bowl with a slotted spoon.

3. In the pot, add the onion, ginger, garlic, and jalapeño pepper and cook for about 4-5 minutes.

4. Press "Cancel" and stir in the beef, spices, and broth.

5. Secure the lid and turn to the "Seal" position.

6. For about 15 minutes cook on "Manual" with "High Pressure".

7. Press "Cancel" and do a "Quick" release.

8. Remove the lid and mix in the carrots.

9. Secure the lid and turn to the "Seal" position.

10. For about 5 minutes cook on "Manual" with "High Pressure".

11. Press "Cancel" and do a "Natural" release for about 10 minutes. Then do a "Quick" release.

12. Remove the lid and mix in the coconut milk.

13. Now, select "Sauté" and cook for about 2-3 minutes.

14. Press "Cancel" and stir in the cilantro.

Nutrition: Calories: 399 | fat: 18.1g | protein: 46.7g | carbs: 10g | net carbs: 7g | fiber: 3g

Pork Lettuce Wraps

Prep Time: 15 minutes

Cook Time: 25 minutes

Serve: 4

Ingredients:

For Pork

- 1 garlic clove, minced finely
- 1 teaspoon dried rosemary
- 1 tablespoon olive oil
- Salt and ground black pepper, to taste
- 1½ pounds pork tenderloin, trimmed and cubed 4 tablespoons water
- 2 tablespoon fresh lemon juice

For Wraps

- ½ cup tomato, chopped finely
- ½ cup cucumber, chopped
- ½ cup onion, chopped
- 2 tablespoons fresh parsley, chopped
- 8 butter lettuce leaves

Instructions:

1. For the pork: Add the garlic, rosemary, oil, salt and black pepper in a wide bowl and mix well.

2. Add the pork and coat with the garlic mixture generously. Set aside for about 15-20 minutes.

3. Place the pork, water, and lemon juice and stir to combine in the pot of Instant Pot.

4. Secure the lid and turn to the "Seal" position.

5. Cook with "High Pressure" on "Manual" for about 25 minutes.

6. Press "Cancel" and do a "Natural" release.

7. Remove the lid and pour the pork into a large bowl with a slotted spoon.

8. With 2 forks, shred the meat.

9. In a bowl, mix together tomato, cucumber, onion, and parsley.

10. Arrange the lettuce leaves onto serving plates.

11. Divide the shredded pork over lettuce leaves evenly and top with tomato mixture.

Nutrition: Calories: 291 | fat: 19.7g | protein: 45.2g | carbs: 3.7g | net carbs: 2.7g | fiber: 1g

Chicken Alfredo Pesto Pasta

Prep time: 10 min

Cook Time: 30 min

Serve: 2

Ingredients:

- ½ pound angel hair pasta, uncooked
- 2 teaspoons oil
- Half kg boneless skinless chicken breasts, cut into bite-size pieces
- 2 cups of milk
- ½ cup PHILADELPHIA Cream Cheese Spread
- 1 large-red-pepper, cut into strips
- ¼ cup KRAFT Grated Parmesan Cheese 2 tablespoons pesto

Instructions:

Cook the pasta omitting salt. Over medium heat, heat oil in a big nonstick skillet. Put chicken and then cook and stir until done or for 7 minutes.

Mix in cream cheese spread and milk. Cook until sauce is well blended and cream cheese is completely melted or for 3 minutes. Put pesto, parmesan and peppers, then stir. Cook until heated through or for 3 minutes, stirring occasionally.

Drain the pasta and place it in the sauce with cream cheese. Coat by tossing it.

Nutrition: Calories 309, Fat 16, Carbs 26, Protein 33, Sodium 755

Chicken Pesto Paninis

Prep time: 10 min

Cook Time: 15 min

Serving: 2

Ingredients:

- 1 focaccia bread, quartered
- 1/2 cup prepared basil pesto
- 1 cup diced cooked chicken
- 1/2 cup diced green bell pepper
- 1/4 cup diced red onion
- 1 cup shredded Monterey Jack cheese

Instructions:

Start preheating a panini grill.

Horizontally cut each quarter of the focaccia bread in half. Spread pesto on each half. Layer equal portions of the chicken, the bell pepper, the onion, and the cheese onto the bottom halves. Place the rest of the focaccia halves on top to have 4 sandwiches.

Place paninis in the prepared grill and grill until cheese is melted and focaccia bread turns golden brown, about 5 minutes.

Nutrition: Calories 350, Fat 12, Carbs 7, Protein 26, Sodium 309

Chicken With Ginger Pesto

Prep time: 10 min

Cook Time: 30 min

Serving: 2

Ingredients:

- 2 pounds skinless, boneless chicken breast halves
- 1/2 cup dry white wine
- 1/4 cup vegetable oil
- 2 little spoons grated fresh ginger root
- 2 cloves garlic_-minced
- 1 littlespoon salt
- 1 littlespoon white sugar
- 1 bunch green onions, cut into 1/4-inch-pieces

Instructions:

1.Combine lightly salted water and wine in a saucepan, place the chicken breasts into the pan. Lower the heat to simmer, bring to a boil, for 8 to 10 minutes until chicken is white and cooked through. Take the chicken out of the sun and let it sit until it cools in the broth. Remove chicken from the broth, set aside.

2.A skillet is placed over medium-low heat, heat vegetable oil, stir in sugar, salt, garlic, and ginger. Cook for about 20 minutes until the garlic is tender and browned and the oil is flavored; remember to stir occasionally when cooking. Stir in green onions, and cook for additional 10 minutes until the onions' white parts are tender; remember to stir occasionally while cooking.

3.Cut poached chicken breasts on the bias into 1 inch wide slices, place decoratively on a plate. Place green onion mixture on top of chicken breasts. Serve.

Nutrition: Calories 584, Fat 21, Carbs 26, Protein 18, Sodium 532

Creamy Pesto Chicken

Prep time: 10 min

Cook Time: 30 min

Serving: 2

Ingredients:

- 1 teaspoon oil
- 4 small boneless skinless chicken breasts
- 1/4 cup PHILADELPHIA Cream Cheese Spread 1/3 cup 25%- less-sodium chicken broth 2 tablespoons pesto

Instructions:

In a big nonstick frying pan, heat oil over medium heat. Put in chicken, cook until done (170°F), or for about 6-8 minutes per side. Remove to a dish; put a cover on to keep warm.

Add cream cheese spread to the frying pan, cook over medium heat until melted, or for about 5 minutes, whisking continually. Mix in pesto and broth, stir and cook until the sauce fully combines and thickens, or for about 2-3 minutes. Add onto the chicken.

Nutrition: Calories 328, Fat 12, Carbs 26, Protein 12, Sodium 459

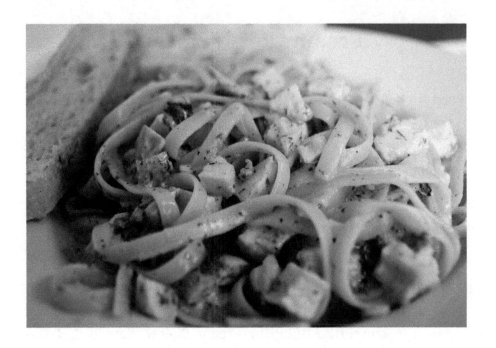

Keto Lobster Roll But With Crab

Prep Time: 20 minutes

Cook Time: 11 minutes

Ingredients:

BUN:

- 1 cup of (100g) almond flour
- 1 scoop (30g) unflavoured whey isolate
- 1.5 tsp of baking powder
- 1 tsp of xanthan gum
- 1/4 cup of melted (50g) butter
- 1/4 cup of (60ml) water
- salt & pepper

"LOBSTER" (crab) SALAD:

- 250g chopped real crab or lobster meat
- 1-2 chopped sticks of celery
- 2-3 chopped green onions
- 1/4 cup of (80g) chopped onions
- 1 tsp of dill
- 1 tsp of minced garlic
- 1/2 cup of (100g) mayonnaise

- Juice from 1/2 a lemon
- A few leaves of lettuce

Instructions:

1. For the buns-combine, all the ingredients in a mixing bowl together until a thick batter forms.

2. Scoop the batter (I used parchment paper to line mine) into greased hot dog bun molds.

3. Wet your hands to make the surface of the dough smooth.

4. Bake for 10-12 minutes at 350 ° F / 175 ° C.

5. Stir all the ingredients for the lobster/crab salad together in a mixing bowl as your buns cook.

6. When the buns are done, let them cool for a few minutes.

7. Like a hot dog bun, slice them open and put a few lettuce leaves in the crack.

8. Fill the lobster/crab salad with it.

Salmon with Veggies

Prep Time: 15 minutes

Cook Time: 6 minutes

Serve: 4

Ingredients:

- 1 pound skin-on salmon fillets
- Salt and ground black pepper, as required
- 1 fresh parsley sprig
- 1 fresh dill sprig
- 3 teaspoons coconut oil, melted and divided ½ lemon, sliced thinly
- 1 carrot, peeled and julienned
- 1 zucchini, peeled and julienned
- 1 red bell pepper, seeded and julienned

Instructions:

1. The salmon fillets are similarly seasoned with salt and black pepper.

2. Arrange a steamer trivet and put herb sprigs and 1 cup of water at the bottom of the Instant Pot.

3. Place the salmon fillets, skin side down on top of the trivet.

4. Drizzle salmon fillets with 2 teaspoons of coconut oil and top with lemon slices.

5. Secure the lid and turn to the "Seal" position.

6. Choose 'Steam' and use the default time of 3 minutes only.

7. Press "Cancel" and do a "Natural" release.

8. Meanwhile, for the sauce: in a bowl, add remaining ingredients and mix until well combined.

9. Remove the lid and transfer the salmon fillets onto a platter.

10. Remove the steamer trivet, herbs, and cooking water from the pot. With paper towels, pat dries the pot.

11. Place the remaining coconut oil in the Instant Pot and select "Sauté". Then add the veggies and cook for about 2-3 minutes.

12. Press "Cancel" and transfer the veggies onto a platter with salmon.

Nutrition: Calories: 204 | fat: 10.6g | protein: 23.1g | carbs: 5.7g | net carbs: 4.3g | fiber: 1.4g

Baked cod with tomatoes and feta

Total time: 30 minutes

Serve: 4

Ingredients:

- 2½ tbsp. olive oil
- 2 garlic cloves
- 2½ cups chopped tomatoes (preferably canned tomatoes with the juice)
- 4 scallions (chopped and separate the white parts from the green parts)
- ¼ tsp. dried oregano
- 12 oz. zucchini
- ½ tsp. salt
- ½ tsp. black pepper
- 1¾ lbs. cod fillet (sliced into 12 pieces)
- 1/3 cup feta cheese
- 1 cup basil (chopped)

Instructions:

1.Take a pan and cook the garlic and the scallions (the white parts) in 1 tbsp. of olive oil until fragrant.

2.Now, add the tomatoes and the oregano and cook them for about 20 minutes, until the tomato sauce gets thicker.

3. In the meantime, the zucchini should be sliced into 1/8-inch thick slices (lengthwise) and, then, put them on the side.

4.When the tomato sauce is thick and ready, remove from heat, put the green parts of the scallions, and stir everything.

5.Preheat the oven to 425°F.

6.Take a tray, arrange the slices of zucchini, and then place the cod on top. Season the cod with ¼ tsp. of black pepper, ½ tsp. of salt, and drizzle with remaining olive oil.

7.Cover the sliced cod with the tomato sauce and the feta cheese. Bake for about 23 minutes, until the cod reaches the temperature of 145°F. When ready, season everything with the chopped basil and the remaining black pepper.

Lightning Source UK Ltd.
Milton Keynes UK
UKHW021258100521
383453UK00001B/45

9 781802 772432